TAKE A
BREAK
BEFORE YOU
BREAK

52
PRACTICAL
SELF-CARE TIPS

Barb –
Take Care –
of Yourself!
All the Best,

By

Breeda Miller

Take a Break Before You Break
52 Practical Self-Care Tips
©2021 by Breeda Miller

Published by Soar 2 Success Publishing

Soar2SuccessPublishing.com

ISBN: 9781943043590

Printed in the United States of America
Photo/Graphics Credit: Lisa Vreede

TABLE OF **CONTENTS**

DEDICATION

This book is dedicated to the givers of the world. Those who give of themselves to care for others, to teach them, lead them, serve them.

One of the most loving acts a giver will do is to care for themselves, so that they may have the strength, resilience, and courage to continue to give of themselves.

To my family for giving me the opportunity to learn and grow in so many different and unexpected ways. Especially, to my beloved husband, Jim, whose constant support and love for nearly four decades has been my foundation.

To our children, Dan, Chloe and Evan, who formed the family we never knew we were meant to be.

NOTE FROM THE AUTHOR

In a perfect world, no one would need a book like this. We would be living our best life doing the things that bring us joy and make the world a better place without neglecting ourselves. But the truth is, few of us have been able to live our lives without becoming overwhelmed and exhausted.

We need to take care of ourselves and that's what this book is about. If you want to be able to be your best self when the going gets rough, you need to have a mindset that will allow you to care for yourself without guilt and without apology.

This book is all about understanding the effect that self-care strategies will have on you and on those with whom you care for and interact. We take better care of our devices than we do ourselves. We need to find ways to be our best selves, and this book will help you do just that.

Breeda Miller

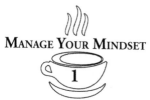

MANAGE YOUR MINDSET

Serenity: What It Is and Isn't

Serenity is not the absence of clamor and commotion,
but the ability to find peace in the midst of it.

The world has changed, and we can waste a lot of time
and energy yearning for the way things used to be.

We will get through this time and finding ways
to become creative and resourceful will make this
time an **opportunity rather than a disaster.**

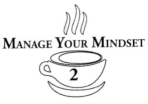

Manage Your Mindset

2

It's a Gratitude Thing

Appreciate life's simple pleasures.
Don't consider what could or should be.
Don't consider what others have or are able to do.

Be mindful and present. What you take for granted
someone else might be eternally grateful for.

A friend broke her leg and sprained her ankle on the other
leg after a bad fall. She has learned what it's like to be
"disabled" in very short order. Even opening doors in the
public bathroom with a walker was nearly impossible.

Realizing that we are all "temporarily abled" can
help you **appreciate all the things you are able
to do** without even thinking about them.

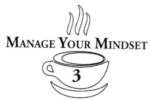

MANAGE YOUR MINDSET

**Sometimes You Need a Pillow.
Sometimes You Are the Pillow.**

Recognize there will be times when you need to ask for help
and support. It's not a sign of weakness. It's a sign of
self-awareness and an opportunity for growth.

It takes a strong and self-confident person to recognize
when they need help, whether it's from a friend or
finding a professional.

Be a resourceful person for your own needs.
When someone else needs help, you will know
what resources are available for them as well.

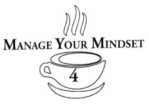

MANAGE YOUR MINDSET

4

Comparison-itis

Know your limits; respect yourself. Just because
your sister is able to scrub a house and cook a
gourmet meal, doesn't mean that you should.

Daily life is not a competition. We often assume that
everyone else has it all figured out and we are the only ones
struggling to get out the door wearing matching shoes.

It's a lie. Everybody has different skills and challenges.
What comes easily for you might bring on migraines
for your colleague. **Don't compare your life to others**,
because you may not have all the information.

Treat everyone you meet as if their heart is breaking because it might be.

4

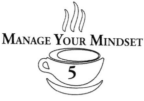

MANAGE YOUR MINDSET

Your Best Self

You can only give away to others what you have inside yourself.

If you are a wreck, physically, mentally and emotionally
you are simply not going to be able to serve others.

Taking time to rest and recharge is not selfish, it's survival.

Problem solving, caring for others, and being
resourceful all take sharp minds and clear heads.

If you really want to be your best self, you
need to take care of yourself.

You need **to be your Best Self**.

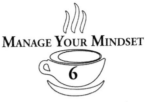

MANAGE YOUR MINDSET

6

Attitude of Gratitude

Gratitude is recognized as an essential component in Good Mental Health. What we focus on, we attract.

Sometimes it's very hard to find the silver lining in challenging circumstances. Times are hard and people are difficult. I often play the game of *It Could Have Been Worse*, and think of how a particular situation could actually have been even more unfortunate.

The current reality then seems more bearable. **Being thankful and showing appreciation** not only enhances your quality of life, but the people around you will also enjoy your presence and the spirit you bring with you.

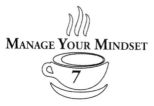

MANAGE YOUR MINDSET

7

Lower your Expectations

Challenging circumstances call for realistic expectations.
It's important to recognize that different situations and life changes
mean that your ability to manage your life will need adjustments.

When you live alone and have only yourself to manage you
can decide the level of cleanliness and organization that works
for you. When you live with others (particularly those with
limited abilities and unlimited needs), you will need to alter
your expectations accordingly. Short cuts, simple meals,
disposable items and unwashed baseboards may be the new
normal. When your sanity and mental health are at **stake, take
all the help you can get and lower your expectations**.

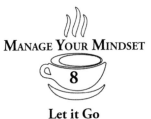

MANAGE YOUR MINDSET

8

Let it Go

Elsa from *Frozen* had it right:
If you can't change it, "Let it go."
We can obsess about our past behavior or mistakes, but it doesn't change anything. If we have wronged someone, we need to make it right. If we have behaved badly, we need to change that behavior. If we simply feel guilty about something in the past and change nothing, it is a waste of time and energy. It prevents us from moving forward.

Guilt can be a great motivator to prevent negative behavior and help us to do the right thing. But, if we live our lives consumed with the guilt of actions or circumstances over which we have no control, we lose the precious time we are given. Do your best; be kind. Correct your mistakes and then
"Let It Go."

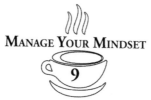

MANAGE YOUR MINDSET

9

An Empty Cup Serves No One

Self-care is not selfish. It's not noble to wear yourself out on behalf of others. You can't be your best self when you are tired, cranky and exhausted. If there is no one looking out for your needs, then you need to step in and take charge. Give yourself permission to rest. Give yourself permission to charge your own battery.

As I've said before, we often take better care of our personal devices than ourselves. Do you begrudge your phone from needing to be charged every night? Of course not! Our phones work hard, and we depend on them. Yet, when we need to take a break, we are often consumed with guilt and just keep pushing ourselves. It's one thing to work hard and do your best. It's quite another thing to burn out and have no reserves left. **"Take a Break Before You Break."**

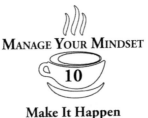

MANAGE YOUR MINDSET
10

Make It Happen

What would you attempt if you knew you couldn't fail? Do you have a dream of the life you'd like to live but dismiss it as impossible? I never thought in a million years that I could walk 200 miles on the Camino de Santiago in Spain at the age of 60. But I did. I have done more things than I ever thought I could do, and I have many more planned.

What would you really like to do that you are holding back on? What can you do to adjust or adapt your dream to make it a reality? I couldn't walk the 500-mile route, but with a slow pace and lots of encouragement I decided to try the 200-mile Portuguese route. It taught me a great lesson.

We are capable of far more than we think. What do you dream of doing? Just take it **one step at a time**.

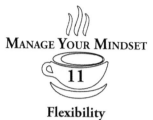

MANAGE YOUR MINDSET

11

Flexibility

Be like Gumby.

Blessed are the flexible for they shall not get bent
out of shape. Adapting to your environment is a sure
way to be more effective and less stressed.

We don't think anything of bundling up in warm clothes when
the weather turns chilly, but when circumstances develop
that require a change in behavior or timing, many find it
hard to adapt. They become rigid and then frustrated.

Particularly when dealing with people who are struggling
with mental or physical health issues, **flexibility is the key to
effective communication,** and ultimately a better outcome.

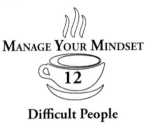

MANAGE YOUR MINDSET

12

Difficult People

One of the most important lessons I have ever learned is this:
If you expect "normal" behavior from a person incapable
of "normal behavior," you will always be disappointed.

Whether it is due to mental illness, addiction, dementia, or other
issues, you are setting yourself up for frustration and unending stress
if you have unrealistic expectations of others. Knowing the person you
are dealing with, their level of understanding and ability to respond
in a logical and reasonable manner, is key to your own mental health.

Remember, *"If you expect normal behavior from*
_____, *you will always be disappointed."*

Act accordingly.

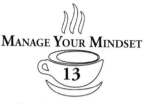

MANAGE YOUR MINDSET

13

Cautious Optimism

When my husband and I were on the Infertility Rollercoaster (not recommended - one star), it was an incredibly stressful time. Each procedure, each month, led to constant disappointment. I learned of a mindset that would help me cope when the outcome was unknown and I had done everything I could.

I would decide to become "Cautiously Optimistic." It allowed me to be hopeful and yet not set myself up for devastation if it didn't end as I planned. This mindset works when you are awaiting test results (of any type), mortgage approval, election results, etc. Our family was created through adoption of three children because we were able to adjust our vision of what our family might look like.

Cautious Optimism is the key.

13

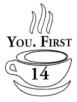

YOU. FIRST

14

Good Shoes and A Soft Path

Take a hike!

I don't mean that in a rude way, of course. But taking a walk can be one of the most restorative things you can do for yourself. It doesn't have to be complicated. Just be sure you are wearing comfortable shoes. I find two pair of socks (for very long hikes) to be really helpful.

There are loads of beautiful natural paths all around us, but just a walk around your neighborhood can provide a wonderful experience. Just get out there.

If you can **find a soft path, a bit of sunshine, lovely shade and a good pair of shoes**, you can't do much better.

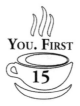

YOU. FIRST

15

Release Tension

You may not even realize it, but your posture
may reflect tension or stress.

Here's a friendly reminder to check that you
are not holding tension in your body.

Let your shoulders drop, unclench your hands and jaw.

Take a deep breath, hold it for few seconds and
let it out slowly.

Aaaaah…. much better.

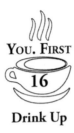

You. First

16

Drink Up

Drink a big glass of water - slowly.

This accomplishes two important things at one time. Dehydration is the source of many physical problems from headaches to urinary tract infections. Drinking a glass of water slowly, also allows an opportunity for mindfulness.

Enjoy the feeling of the glass (pick a nice one), the coolness and condensation. Sip the water and feel it in your mouth. Take your time swallowing it.

You can really drag this out and make it a simple, yet effective break in your day. **A big glass of fresh water provides a welcome, wet respite** several times a day. Give it a try and drink up.

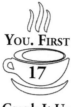

You. First

17

Crank It Up

In your car, crank up the jams. A dear friend told me that when she is feeling really stressed and needs to get away from everybody, she gets in her car, rolls UP the windows and blasts her favorite tunes on the radio.

With *Spotify*, *Apple Music*, *Pandora* or just your *own playlist* on your phone, you can choose to rock out to *Motown*, *The Beatles*, *Bon Jovi*, *Nickelback (jk!)*, *Elvis*, *Garth Brooks* or *Broadway soundtracks*.

It can be exhilarating and so much fun. Plan your own selfie concert in your driveway soon.

Enjoy a musical break just for you!

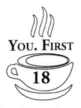

YOU. FIRST

18

Plan Your Escape

Take 10 minutes and plan your fantasy getaway.
This is where *Pinterest* can really be your friend. Create a
*collection of beautiful locations, favorite foods, grand adventures
and majestic scenes.* As you take time to sort and save your
favorites, imagine yourself right inside the photo. You can take
it a step further and find foods and drinks that connect with
your fantasy escape and enjoy it right at home right now.

The world is experiencing travel restrictions and you may
have your own restrictions due to family responsibilities
and finances, but that doesn't mean you can't **enjoy a
mental escape.** Add to this by finding a good book set in
the location you are thinking about to immerse yourself in
even more details: ***BreedaMiller.com/favoriteplaces***

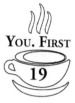

You. First

19

Reading for Fun

Reading for pleasure is such a novel thing to do.

See what I did there? Truly, taking the time to find a good
book (or even a trashy one) to escape with can be a luxurious
retreat and it can expand your horizons at a time when
our world can seem exceedingly small and limited.

Make sure you have a comfy spot to read with good lighting.
Maybe it's your couch, a favorite chair, or even a
cozy window seat with loads of pillows.

Give yourself permission to read something that
isn't academic or related to your work.

You will give yourself the world

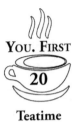

YOU. FIRST

20

Teatime

Be intentional.

Set up a time and place. Make it an event.

Whether it's herbal, black or green, flavored or
traditional, make it a moment to savor.

Brew the tea; maybe even use a nice small teapot. Drink it from
a favorite cup or mug and take the time to sit and savor.

My mom used to say that *tea solves most of the
problems of the world, at least for a few minutes.*

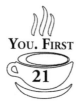

YOU. FIRST

21

Find Your People

Finding people who share a common interest can be challenging, depending on where you live and your circumstances. But sharing a hobby, an interest or a talent with a social group can greatly improve your quality of life.

It can provide you with a structure to **"Take A Break"** as well an opportunity for social interaction. Whether it's an online community or an in-person gathering, putting yourself out there can open up a world of opportunity and fun.

Types of groups to consider: *Travel, sports, collections, faith, crafts, art, books, games, environment, community support.*

There are as many special interests as there are people. **Step outside and find your people.**

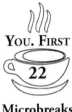

You, First

22

Microbreaks

Sometimes the idea of *Taking a Break* is just overwhelming. It might feel like it's just not possible or too much work. It's true that planning a much-deserved vacation or a workout at the gym takes planning. But what about planning Microbreaks in your day?

For five or ten minutes every day, plan something that you can anticipate and enjoy. Simple is best, whether it be a brisk walk around the block, savoring your coffee in a favorite mug, reading a few chapters of a juicy novel, or sitting outside and taking deep breaths. Just be sure it is intentional and in a slightly different location than your working environment. A little break can go a long way.

More at BreedaMiller.com/breedatv

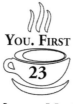

YOU. FIRST

23

Massage Magic

I'm embarrassed to admit how old I was
before I had my first massage.

I was intimidated and had no idea what it was all about.

The good news is that I got over my embarrassment
and credit a monthly massage with keeping my
sanity when I was my mother's caregiver.

It's the best gift ever and you can give it to yourself.

One size fits all and there is no need to put it away or dust it.

Who could ask for more?

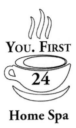

You. First

24

Home Spa

Give yourself the gift of a little pampering.

Dig out the goodies you've received and set
up your own home spa one evening.

Put on a comfy robe, fuzzy slippers (yes, you fellas too),
fill a tub with a foot soak, take a bubble bath, use that
fancy facial mask, and maybe even polish your nails.

You don't need a special occasion or a lot of money to
find a bit of luxury.

Make a date with yourself for a little spa at home.

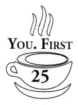

YOU. FIRST

25

Low Tech Organization

Peace of mind is a wonderful gift to give yourself and your family. Create accessible files for family/business with essential information available for those who need it if you are not available.

Low tech solutions can really come in handy during power outages or when passwords are a mystery to everyone else but you. Old fashioned binders with clear plastic sleeves are a great solution. Each family member should have one with their key personal documents stored inside. You can also create a binder just for important document categories like automobiles, insurance, and pets. You can make it as simple or elaborate as you like, but it will **allow your family to find what they need when they need it most.**

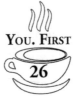

YOU. FIRST

26

Annoying Noise

This is a remarkably simple thing, but it can make a huge difference in your daily life. Banish annoying ring tones and alarms that surround you. Take a few minutes and think about your phone sounds. Do they annoy you? Can you hear them? Are they too loud?

Maybe it would be fun to have your favorite song or one that takes you back to a moment in time to be your ring tone. Maybe it's an uplifting tune or something silly that makes you smile. My daughter has the sound of crickets as her alarm sound on her phone. My ring tone is the Harry Potter theme and every time it rings in public, people smile. It makes me smile and it's an easy thing to do.
Remove the annoying sounds in your life. It's a little thing that just makes life a bit more pleasant.

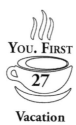

You. First

27

Vacation

The ultimate "break" is taking a vacation. We all need a vacation, now more than ever. If you are unable to just pick up and go, there is also great benefit in plotting and planning a break away from your regular routine. Dreaming of a destination, considering the options, and determining which is the best one is a break in itself.

Whether you like to camp in a local state park or fly to a far-off land, the anticipation of a trip is half the fun. Family responsibilities mean you need to take more details into consideration, but it still may be possible. Ask for help, give people notice, and you might be surprised at the positive responses you receive. Even a day trip can be refreshing and rejuvenating. You just must make it happen.

We all need a break, and you deserve it.

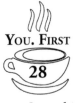

You. First

28

Create Something

Mental and emotional stress will exhaust you.

Sometimes the best way to take a break is to
create something. Consider taking an old piece of
furniture and turning it into something new.

The physical activity of sanding wood, painting something old and
making it look fresh and new is not only a satisfying expression
of creativity, the physical release from hammering, sanding,
and painting will provide a wonderful break for your brain and
all the thinking and worrying that you have been carrying.

The bonus is that you will have something to **make
your space more personal and comfortable.**

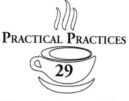

PRACTICAL PRACTICES

29

Never Exchange Gifts

Be a giver.

*When you give cheerfully and accept gracefully, everyone is blessed - **Maya Angelou**.*

When you exchange gifts, it is a transaction rather than a moment of blessing. Find a way to give to others without expecting anything in return.

When you accept a gift graciously, you are giving a gift to the person who gifted you. No apologies, no explanations. A sincere thank you and a big smile are wonderful gifts.

Take pressure off yourself to have an equal exchange. That's a transaction.

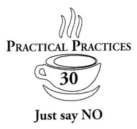

PRACTICAL PRACTICES

30

Just say NO

You are not the general manager of the universe.
You can only truly control yourself and the way you respond
to people and situations. This is a tough one for many
people. You really don't have to be, nor can you truly be,
responsible for everyone and everything. It's an unrealistic
expectation and sets you up for exhaustion and frustration.

Remember, the word NO is a complete sentence. One of my
favorite ways to say no to an invitation or an opportunity
that I don't want to engage in is to say, "*Thanks, but it's not
for me.*" Full stop; no further explanation is required.

**Give yourself permission to say no to things
that don't serve you.**

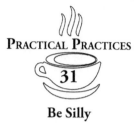

PRACTICAL PRACTICES

31

Be Silly

Don't feel obligated to act your age.

One of the best things about having kids or grandkids is that you have a legitimate excuse to build a blanket fort or go to the zoo. But if you don't have these little people in your life, there is no reason that you can't find silly ways to have fun.

Is there a craft or artistic project you've always wanted to explore? How about a day at an amusement park? When was the last time you blew bubbles with a little round wand?

Finding joy in simple, silly things is a great way to release some pressure.

Being an adult is hard. "Take a Break."

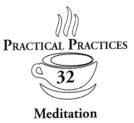

PRACTICAL PRACTICES

32

Meditation

I've never been one to have the discipline to meditate regularly or even irregularly. However, when I have taken the time, I have found that using an app or a video on YouTube was a tremendous help.

It's like a **mini vacation** - often only 10 or 15 minutes in length. There are some really fabulous programs that are free. It's worth your time to sample a few and decide if they will work for you. The Calm App is free, and I also like the *21 Day programs with Deepak Chopra*.

It's worth a try and it can make a huge difference.

My blog has more thoughts on meditation:
BreedaMiller.com/calmyourmind

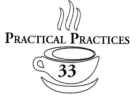

PRACTICAL PRACTICES

33

Permission Granted

As a leader, it can be hard to give yourself permission to pause, to take a break. If that has been a challenge for you, I hereby grant you permission to take a break.

You will not only be doing something really good for yourself, but you will also be setting a healthy example for your team and members of your family.

We lead by example.

A leader who is able to find balance by taking the time to recharge, replenish and refresh will earn respect and be appreciated.

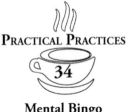

PRACTICAL PRACTICES
34

Mental Bingo

Playing "Mental Bingo" is one of my favorite coping strategies. Whenever things that people say or do repeatedly get on my nerves, I award them (secretly) a spot on my Mental Bingo card. Then when they do the thing that I know they are going to do, or say the words that get under my skin, I silently check off that box on my "Mental Bingo" card.

When they've done it five times, I get to say BINGO! It's strangely satisfying and bit of silly fun. I realize I can't change their actions or words, but I can control my response to it. I can refuse to allow it to control me and affect my attitude in a negative way. That space in my brain is precious real estate and I'm not giving it away to anyone. **"Mental Bingo" helps.**

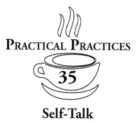

PRACTICAL PRACTICES

35

Self-Talk

Imagine you are speaking to someone very dear to you. You can see they are disheartened, frustrated, or upset.

What would you say to them? What tone would you use? Would you wag your finger at them?

You might be gentle and listen. You might be supportive and kind. You might offer them consolation. Why would you not do that for yourself?

No one can be more dear or precious to you than your own spirit, never at the expense of others of course, but as an example of true love. Make sure the words you say to yourself help you to "**Be Better, not Bitter.**"

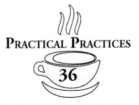

PRACTICAL PRACTICES
36

Build your Own Bubble

A lesson from COVID-19: Decide who is in your bubble.
In 2020, we experienced a pandemic that turned our
world upside down. All the activities we took for granted
were now a logistical and physical challenge.

Where can we go? Who can we see? What can we do?
Just as staying safe during a pandemic requires careful planning,
living a healthy life during ordinary times means setting
boundaries and making choices. Who is toxic in your life? Who
is too big a risk? Who might cause harm? Taking care of yourself
means surrounding yourself with people you enjoy and who
care about you as much as you care about them. Being with the
right person is not a guarantee of happiness but being with the
wrong person is an opportunity for misery. **Choose wisely.**

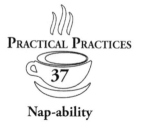

PRACTICAL PRACTICES

37

Nap-ability

Is there anything as delicious as an afternoon nap in a comfy spot? What is your nap-ability? Not everyone has this skill but if you have it, I hope you honor and cherish it for the gift that it is. You can increase your ability to take a refreshing nap by setting yourself up for success.

Here are a few tips from the experts: Choose a spot that is comfortable and quiet. Use an eye mask to block out light. Set an alarm on your phone so you don't worry about oversleeping. Imagine your body sinking deeply into the couch or chair. Count slowly and start relaxing your feet, your legs, your hands, your arms, and your torso. Give yourself 15 minutes. **Even if you don't actually fall asleep you will feel a benefit from this experience.**

37

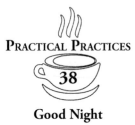

PRACTICAL PRACTICES

38

Good Night

Getting a good night's sleep is essential. If this is a challenge
for you, here are some tips to send you into dreamland.

- Splurge on good sheets. They are a luxury you will enjoy every
  night.
- Avoid eating 2-3 hours before bedtime. It's harder for your
  body to wind down when it's busy digesting food.
- Use caffeine wisely. (Remember that soda and tea can contain
  caffeine.)
- Take a warm bath or shower before bed to help you relax.
- Room darkening shades or a sleep mask can help in the
  summer months.
- Keep away from the blue light on your devices and TV.
- Fill your mind with the three things for which you are grateful.

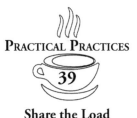

PRACTICAL PRACTICES

39

Share the Load

Delegating can be really hard and it takes trust to do it well.

You may feel obligated to do everything for everyone.

That is simply not realistic and it denies others the opportunity to learn and be part of your world.

The time is takes to explain and teach someone how they can participate and contribute is well worth it.

You will be able to "Take a Break" and know that the world will keep turning and life can go on without you for a bit.

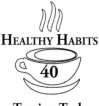

HEALTHY HABITS
40

Taming Tech

Consider the technology in your life. What serves
you? What stresses you? How can you change what
depletes your energy or your effectiveness?

Now that so many of us are working from home, it can be hard
to communicate easily. Now we send an email to set up a time
for a phone call or a Zoom call. How about a day that you
intentionally reach out to friends for just for a little chat and
connection? Make a date with yourself and make it happen.

You tame the tech; don't let it control you. Remember, you
don't have to answer every call. Angela from the extended
warranty department will be fine without you.

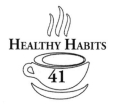

HEALTHY HABITS

41

When Less is a Lot More

Do you feel like you are a hamster on a wheel,
constantly in motion but never getting anywhere?

What can you stop doing that will move
you forward and reduce your stress?

What can you do differently or what resources can you find
that can help you actually do less and accomplish more?

Be productive; do a little less.

Focus, plan and recharge to make things happen.
Consider how you spend your 24 hours.
Here's a worksheet to help you: ***BreedaMiller.com/hamster***

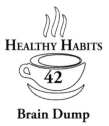

HEALTHY HABITS

42

Brain Dump

Trying to remember everything and keep it all straight is a huge burden on your brain. As you lie in bed at night, you may second guess your actions and try to remember what still needs to be done.

Write it all down. Call it a brain dump, a master to-do list, or simply your hopes and dreams. It will be one of the best things you can do for your peace of mind. It is incredibly satisfying to see a list and be able to check off items.

One system that is especially helpful is the ***Bullet Journal*** method. It's a way of organizing your to do lists with your dreams and special projects, enabling you to make it happen. Check more details here: ***BreedaMiller.com/bulletjournal***

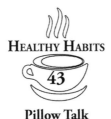

HEALTHY HABITS

43

Pillow Talk

When you finally lay your head down on your pillow what thoughts fill your mind? Are they all the regrets of the day? What you should've, could've done? All the tasks still left to do?

Instead, fill your mind and your heart with three things that will help you relax and crowd out those negative and stressful thoughts:

1. Something that you are grateful for.
2. Something that went better than you had expected.
3. Something that you are looking forward to (no matter how far in the future).

Sleep well. It's a break that is essential.

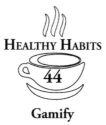

HEALTHY HABITS

44

Gamify

Many of us spend too much time attached to our phones and that can have a negative impact on our mindset.

But zoning out and playing some mindless games can be a healthy little escape right in the palm of your hand.

Solitaire, CandyCrush, Bubbles or cat games - are simple relaxing video games on your phone. The key thing about these games is to manage the time you spend with them and not let them have a negative impact.

When anxiety creeps up and you need a simple distraction, these **little games might just do the trick**.

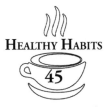

HEALTHY HABITS

45

Anti-stress Foods

We all know what our favorite comfort foods are, though
they may not be the best anti-stress choices.

If you are interested in choosing some anti-stress foods to
help you Take a Break, here are some good options:

- Fruit, Vegetables and Berries: Avocado (my fave), leafy greens
  and blackberries
- Nuts and Seeds: Pistachio, Pumpkin, Sesame and Sunflower
- Meats: Turkey and Salmon
- Treats: Dark Chocolate

Keep these handy and find ways to include them in
your meals. **They're good and good for you**.

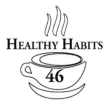

HEALTHY HABITS

46

Rituals and Routines

Creating intentional rituals and routines make self-care a natural part of your life, rather than a special occasion. Build into your day healthy habits that will make you feel better, like drinking lots of water, getting outside, moving more and eating healthy food. But also give yourself permission to listen to your body.

When you need to rest and slow down, do it. Take five or ten minutes and find a quiet spot to close your eyes and put your feet up. Recognizing signs of exhaustion is not a weakness, it's honoring your body and your spirit. Self-care isn't selfish, it's survival. I'd love to hear your healthy habits. Go to ***BreedaMiller.com/wildside*** and comment. I read each one!

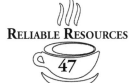

RELIABLE RESOURCES

47

Podcasts

I'm fairly late to the party on this, but I have
fallen in love with listening to Podcasts.

There is a such a wide variety of these little gems to make your
commute or walk a time of relaxation, entertainment,
or education.

You can learn techniques and strategies, be entertained with
stories, and understand other points of view. Someone has
created a podcast for just about any topic you are interested in.

They're **free and fabulous**. Not sure where to start? Go
to *BreedaMiller.com/resources* to see a list of mine.

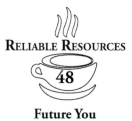

RELIABLE RESOURCES

48

Future You

Never underestimate the value of a first-floor bathroom and bedroom. It's easy enough to create a temporary bedroom on the first floor in an emergency situation.

That second-floor bathroom is often a deal breaker and prevents many people from staying in their own homes as long as they would like.

Consider your own needs and those of your parents as you make decisions regarding homes and accessibility. Those stairs may not be problem now, but if someday you have to have a knee replaced you might have a different opinion.

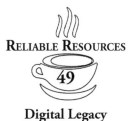

RELIABLE RESOURCES

49

Digital Legacy

If you're the keeper of family photos, documents and
treasured stories, there is a great way to share them
with family and remove the burden of owning these
things. Create a **digital book of your family**.
You can find a platform that will allow you build a legacy and
then share it with your family. This will become a treasure and
you can get a hard copy printed as well. I used Blurb.com and it's
free until you decide to print a copy. I selected the largest format
and a simple background. You can get your photos scanned
at a variety of businesses and there is no deadline to finish.
Doing this will be a gift to yourself as you release the burden of
what to do with all these photos and treasured documents.
Go to *BreedaMiller.com/digital-legacy* for
more details about how to do this.

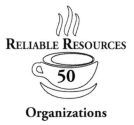

RELIABLE RESOURCES

50

Organizations

There are wonderful organizations that are available to support you, whether it's a temporary stressor or long-term situation. You don't have to figure it out alone.

National organizations often have state or local chapters that can provide incredible connections and information.

Do you need support in dealing with an illness or solving a problem? Do you want to develop a new skill or start a new profession? Are you interested in connecting with other people interested in similar things or ideas? **Your people are out there.**

For more information visit *BreedaMiller.com/resources*

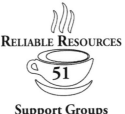

RELIABLE RESOURCES

51

Support Groups

If you are dealing with an illness or physical challenge,
or if you are caring for someone who has special needs,
there seems to be support group for just about
everything and everyone.

I have created a long list of support groups on
BreedaMiller.com/Resources. If your special need
is not listed here, just Google the name of your need
and support group and you'll likely find help.

Please let me know of support groups that may help
others. Drop me a line at ***Breeda@BreedaMiller.com***

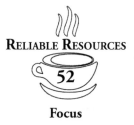

RELIABLE RESOURCES

52

Focus

When you need to complete an important task, consider music as an assistant. I found a playlist on Spotify that really helps my brain focus and get into the flow.

It's called *Focus on Spotify* and it's free. You can set a timer and just dive in with your earbuds in and tune the world out.

Many people use the *Pomodoro method*, which is simply setting a timer for a certain length of time (like 25 minutes) and working without taking any sort of break.

Fun Fact: The Pomodoro method was named because the timer that was used was a red plastic tomato and Pomodoro means tomato in Italian. Sounds much fancier than the Tomato Method.

NOTE FROM BREEDA MILLER

I hope you have enjoyed ***Take A Break Before You Break*** and that you have discovered ideas and strategies that will help you help others because you will be able to take time to care for yourself.

If your organization is looking for in-person or virtual programs that expand on the tips in this book, I'd be delighted to chat with you. I have also created a special video series called **CareBoost** that provides short messages with big impact.

To learn more about working with me, please visit my website, ***BreedaMillerSpeaking.com***.

NEED A SPEAKER?

Breeda Miller Speaking provides organizations with a variety of services. Whether you are looking for an engaging and entertaining keynote speaker or an interactive break out session, Breeda Miller is ready to work with you. As a professional member of the *National Speakers Association*, and past president of the *Michigan Chapter of NSA*, Breeda has the expertise and the experience to make your event one worth attending.

A Certified Virtual Presenter as well as nationally recognized storyteller is a phenomenal combination to ensure the success of your next event. Contact Breeda to find out how she can serve your needs.

Email Breeda: ***Breeda@ Breedamiller.com*** or go to:
BreedaMillerSpeaking.com

ABOUT BREEDA MILLER

An author, speaker, and trainer, Breeda Miller has used her professional experience serving clients in health care organizations, corporations, academic institutions, and non-profit communities.

Apart from her education, Breeda came to her awareness of the value of self-care when she cared for her mother for nearly six years, including hospice care in her home.

She is a graduate of the University of Detroit Mercy and has a variety of certifications and training programs.

A skilled storyteller, her video stories have gone viral and she has appeared on *The Moth Story Hour* on NPR.

Through the power of story, audience interaction and warm-hearted humor, Breeda presents strategies that make a difference.

CONNECT WITH BREEDA

BreedaMiller.com
BreedaMillerSpeaking.com
Breeda@Breedamiller.com

OTHER BOOKS BY BREEDA

The Caregiver Coffeebreak –
76 practical tips to Help Caregivers Take a Break
A warm-hearted tip book supporting family and
professional caregivers

SOCIAL MEDIA

Facebook.com/BreedaMiller
Twitter.com/BreedaMiller
LinkedIn.com/in/BreedaMiller
YouTube/BreedaTV.com